The 90-Day Transformation: A Quick Guide to Fitness, Nutrition, and Lasting Change

Table of Contents

Chapter 1: The Importance of 90 Days - Setting the Stage for Success

• Understanding the science behind habit formation and why 90 days is the ideal timeframe

• The psychology of transformation: mindset shifts for long-term success

• Setting realistic and achievable goals for your 90-day journey

• The importance of tracking progress and celebrating small wins

• Introduction to the "Momentum Method" for maintaining motivation

Chapter 2: Crafting Your Personalized 90-Day Fitness Plan

• Assessing your current fitness level and setting suitable benchmarks

• Balancing strength training, cardio, and flexibility work

• Designing workouts for different fitness goals (weight loss, muscle gain, toning)

• Incorporating HIIT for most fat burning and time efficiency

• Adapting exercises for home, gym, or outdoor settings

• Progressive overload: The key to continuous improvement

• Injury prevention strategies for intense 90-day programs

Chapter 3: Nutrition Fundamentals for Optimal Results

• Calculating your ideal calorie intake for your specific goals

• Macronutrient balance: Finding your perfect protein, carbohydrates, and fat ratio

• The truth about "good" and "bad" carbs: Dispelling common myths

• Essential micronutrients for health and performance

• Hydration strategies for enhanced metabolism and recovery

• The "Plate Method" for easy meal planning and portion control

• Navigating food labels and making informed choices

Chapter 4: Meal Planning and Prep for Success

• Creating a sustainable 90-day meal plan tailored to your preferences

• Grocery shopping tips for staying on track and on budget

• Batch cooking and meal prep strategies to save time and reduce stress

• Quick and healthy recipes for breakfast, lunch, dinner, and snacks

• Dealing with cravings and emotional eating during your transformation

• Eating out and social situations: How to stay on plan without sacrificing your social life

• The "Flexible Five" approach to incorporating treats without derailing progress

Chapter 5: Supercharging Fat Loss: Advanced Strategies

• The science of fat burning: Understanding how your body loses fat

• Targeted exercises for stubborn areas (belly, thighs, arms)

• The role of sleep in fat loss and how to optimize your sleep routine

• Stress management techniques to reduce cortisol and promote fat burning

• Intermittent fasting: Is it right for you? Pros, cons, and implementation

• Supplements that can aid fat loss (and which ones to avoid)

• The surprising link between gut health and weight loss

Chapter 6: Building Lean Muscle Mass in 90 Days

• The biology of muscle growth and how to optimize it

• Essential exercises for each major muscle group

• Proper form and technique to maximize muscle activation

• Nutrition strategies for muscle gain without excessive fat gain

• The importance of rest and recovery in muscle building

• Breaking through plateaus with advanced training techniques

• Body composition: How to build muscle and lose fat simultaneously

Chapter 7: Boosting Cardiovascular Health and Endurance

• Understanding the different types of cardio and their benefits

• Designing a progressive cardio plan for improved heart health

• Interval training for most cardiovascular benefits

• Incorporating functional movements for real-world fitness

• Breathing techniques to enhance endurance and performance

• Monitoring heart rate and using heart rate zones effectively

• The unexpected benefits of improved cardiovascular health on overall well-being

Chapter 8: Flexibility, Mobility, and Injury Prevention

• The often-overlooked importance of flexibility in overall fitness

• Dynamic stretching routines for pre-workout preparation

• Static stretching and its role in recovery and injury prevention

• Yoga and Pilates: Incorporating mind-body practices into your routine

• Foam rolling and self-massage techniques for muscle recovery

• Corrective exercises to address common imbalances and prevent injury

• The "Prehab Protocol" for bulletproofing your body against common fitness injuries

Chapter 9: Nutrition Deep Dive: Fueling Your Transformation

• The role of protein in muscle building and recovery

• Carbohydrates: Timing and types for optimal performance

• Healthy fats and their impact on hormones and overall health

• Pre- and post-workout nutrition for most results

• The truth about detoxes and cleanses: What works and what does not

• Navigating dietary restrictions (vegan, gluten-free, etc.) within your plan

• Supplements: What's worth it and what's a waste of money

Chapter 10: Mind-Body Connection: Mental Strategies for Success

• The power of visualization in achieving fitness goals

• Developing a positive body image throughout your transformation

• Mindfulness and meditation practices for stress reduction and focus

• Overcoming mental barriers and self-sabotaging behaviors

• The role of sleep in mental health and physical performance

• Building resilience and grit for long-term success

• The "Mental Momentum Method" for pushing through tough days

Chapter 11: Lifestyle Integration: Making Your 90-Day Plan Sustainable

• Balancing fitness goals with work and family commitments

• Creating a supportive environment for success

• Strategies for staying on track during travel and vacations

• Dealing with unsupportive friends or family members

• Incorporating active hobbies for enjoyable fitness

• The importance of rest and recovery in a sustainable plan

• Planning for life after the 90 days: Transitioning to long-term habits

Chapter 12: Tracking Progress and Adjusting Your Plan

• Beyond the scale: Comprehensive methods for measuring progress

• Using progress photos, measurements, and fitness tests effectively

• The pros and cons of body fat measurement techniques

• When and how to adjust your plan based on results

• Dealing with plateaus: Strategies to reignite progress

• The importance of non-scale victories in motivation

• Creating a personal dashboard for holistic progress tracking

Chapter 13: Special Considerations for Different Populations

• Adapting the 90-day plan for seniors: Focus on functional fitness and bone health

• Postpartum fitness: Safe and effective strategies for new mothers

• Managing chronic conditions through diet and exercise

• Fitness strategies for shift workers and irregular schedules

• Adapting the plan for different body types and genetic factors

• Addressing hormonal changes: Plans for menopause and andropause

• Modifications for people who have limited mobility or chronic pain

Chapter 14: The Role of Technology in Your 90-Day Journey

• Choosing the right fitness tracker or smartwatch for your goals

• Apps and software for meal planning and tracking

• Virtual personal training and online coaching options

• Using social media for accountability and support

• The pros and cons of AI-powered fitness plans

• Leveraging technology for proper form and technique

• Privacy considerations when using fitness tech

Chapter 15: Beyond 90 Days: Maintaining Your Transformation

• Transitioning from a structured plan to sustainable lifestyle habits

• Strategies for maintaining motivation without a specific end date

• Adjusting your nutrition plan for maintenance vs. continued progress

• The importance of periodization in long-term fitness plans

• Setting new goals and challenges to keep progress exciting

• Dealing with setbacks and getting back on track quickly

• The "Lifestyle Integration Method" for permanent change

Appendix A: Quick Reference 90-Day Workout Plans for Different Goals

Appendix B: Progress Tracking Sheets and Journals

Chapter 1: The Importance of 90 Days - Setting the Stage for Success

Imagine the incredible transformation you could achieve in just 90 days. Science has proven that this timeframe is the sweet spot for creating lasting habits and making significant progress towards your fitness and nutrition goals. By committing to a 90-day journey, you set the stage for success and create your potential for long-term, sustainable change. The power of 90 days comes from the psychology of habit formation. Research shows that it takes an average of 66 days for a new behavior to become automatic, but 90 days provides a buffer to solidify your new habits and make them stick.

During this time, your brain rewires itself, forming new neural pathways that support your desired behaviors, making them feel more natural and efficient over time. To maximize your 90-day transformation, start by adopting a growth mindset. Embrace challenges as opportunities for learning and improvement, and view setbacks as temporary obstacles to overcome. This shift in perspective will help you stay resilient and committed, even when the journey gets tough.

Setting realistic and achievable goals is crucial for your 90-day success. Break down your ultimate vision into smaller, manageable milestones that you can work towards each week or month. This approach keeps you motivated and allows you to celebrate the small wins along the way, reinforcing your progress and building momentum. Remember, the key to 90-Day Success: Track, Celebrate, and Maintain Momentum.

Tracking your progress is essential for staying accountable and motivated throughout your 90-day journey. Keep a journal, use a fitness app, or take progress photos to visually document your transformation. Regularly reviewing your progress will help you stay focused on your goals and make adjustments as needed.

Celebrating your small wins is just as important as tracking your progress. Acknowledge your achievements, no matter how small they may seem, and reward yourself for your hard work. This positive reinforcement will keep you motivated and remind you of how far you have come.

To maintain your motivation throughout the 90 days, embrace the "Momentum Method." This approach involves consistently taking action, no matter how small, to keep your progress moving forward. Even on days when you do not feel like working out or eating healthily, commit to doing something, like a 10-minute walk or choosing a nutritious snack. These small actions add up over time and help you maintain your momentum.

Remember, your 90-day journey is not about perfection, but rather about progress. Embrace the challenges, learn from your setbacks, and celebrate your victories along the way. By committing to this transformative timeframe, you will achieve your fitness and nutrition goals and develop the habits and mindset necessary for long-term success. As you set off on your 90-day journey, keep this powerful quote from Aristotle in mind: "We are what we repeatedly do.

Chapter 2: Crafting Your Personalized 90-Day Fitness Plan

You have made the commitment to improve your body and health over the next 90 days. Congratulations on taking this crucial first step! Now, it is time to design a fitness plan tailored to your unique goals, preferences, and lifestyle. By strategically combining strength training, cardio, and flexibility work, you will be well on your way to achieving the physique you have always wanted.

Start by assessing your current fitness level. This will help you set realistic benchmarks and track your progress along the way. Consider factors such as your body composition, cardiovascular endurance, and strength in various muscle groups. Do not worry if you are not where you want to be just yet – that is what this 90-day journey is all about!

When crafting your plan, aim for a balance of strength training, cardio, and flexibility work. The specific ratio will depend on your primary goal, whether it is fat loss, muscle gain, or overall toning. For fat loss, focus on high-intensity interval training (HIIT) and compound strength exercises that target multiple muscle groups simultaneously. If you are looking to build muscle, prioritize resistance training with progressively heavier weights and plenty of rest between workouts. And if toning is your main goal, combine moderate weights with higher repetitions and shorter rest periods.

HIIT deserves special attention in your 90-day plan due to its unparalleled fat-burning potential and time efficiency. By alternating short bursts of all-out effort with brief recovery periods, you will keep your metabolism revved up for hours after each workout. Incorporate HIIT sessions into your cardio routine two to three times per week, using exercises like sprints, burpees, or jumping jacks.

"The only bad workout is the one that didn't happen." – Unknown. Remember, consistency is key. Design your workouts to fit seamlessly into your schedule and preferences. If you love the outdoors, plan invigorating trail runs or park bench workouts. If you thrive on gym equipment, build routines around the machines and free weights available. And if home workouts are most convenient, invest in a few versatile pieces like resistance bands and a stability ball. The more enjoyable and accessible your workouts are, the more likely you will be to stick with them.

As you progress through your 90-day plan, embrace the concept of progressive overload. Gradually increase the intensity, duration, or frequency of your workouts to keep your body challenged and avoid plateaus. This could mean adding an extra set to your strength routine, shaving seconds off your HIIT intervals, or holding your yoga poses for a few breaths longer. By continually pushing your limits, you will ensure ongoing progress and results.

Of course, with intense training comes the need for proper recovery and injury prevention. Schedule regular rest days and prioritize sleep to allow your muscles time to repair and grow. Incorporate dynamic stretching before workouts and static stretching afterwards to maintain flexibility and minimize the risk of strains or sprains. And do not hesitate to change exercises or reduce intensity if you experience pain or excessive fatigue. Your 90-day journey is a marathon, not a sprint – pace yourself accordingly.

Key Takeaways:

- Assess your current fitness level and set realistic benchmarks

- Balance strength training, cardio, and flexibility work based on your primary goal

- Incorporate HIIT for maximum fat burning and time efficiency

- Design workouts that fit your schedule, preferences, and available equipment

- Embrace progressive overload to avoid plateaus and ensure ongoing progress

- Prioritize recovery and injury prevention through rest, sleep, and proper stretching

With a personalized plan in place, you are ready to begin on your 90-day transformation.

Chapter 3: Nutrition Fundamentals for Optimal Results

You have committed to your fitness journey, and now it is time to fuel your body for optimal results. Nutrition is the foundation of your success, and in this chapter, we will dive into the fundamentals that will empower you to make informed choices and create a sustainable eating plan tailored to your unique goals. Picture your body as a high-performance vehicle. Just as a car requires the right type and amount of fuel to run efficiently, your body needs the proper balance of nutrients to function at its best.

The first step in optimizing your nutrition is calculating your ideal calorie intake based on factors such as your age, gender, height, weight, and activity level. This personalized approach confirms that you are providing your body with the energy it needs to support your fitness goals, whether you aim to lose fat, build muscle, or maintain your current physique. A general formula to calculate this number for women is 655 + (4.35 x weight in pounds) + 4.7 x height in inches) –(4.7 x age), and for men 66 +(6.23 x weight in pounds) + (12.7 x height in inches)-(6.8 x age). Depending on your activity level, this number should then be multiplied by 1.2 if sedentary, 1.375 if lightly active, 1.55 if moderately active, 1.725 if very active, and 1.9 if extra active.

Next, let us explore the concept of macronutrient balance. Macronutrients—protein, carbohydrates, and fat—are the essential building blocks of your diet. Finding the right ratio of these nutrients is crucial for supporting your training, recovery, and overall health. While there is no one-size-fits-all approach, a general guideline is to aim for a balance of lean proteins, complex carbohydrates, and healthy fats at each meal. Experiment with different ratios and listen to your body's feedback to find out about your optimal macronutrient mix.

When it comes to carbohydrates, it is time to dispel some common myths. You may have heard that carbs are the enemy, but the truth is more nuanced. Quality matters more than quantity. Focus on consuming nutrient-dense, whole-food sources of carbohydrates such as fruits, vegetables, whole grains, and legumes. These "good" carbs provide essential vitamins, minerals, and fiber that support your health and energy levels. On the other hand, limit your intake of refined, processed carbs like sugary snacks and white bread, which can lead to energy crashes and hinder your progress.

In addition to macronutrients, micronutrients play a vital role in your overall health and performance. Essential vitamins and minerals such as iron, calcium, magnesium, and B vitamins support various bodily functions, from bone health to energy production. Ensure that your diet includes a colorful array of fruits and vegetables to get a wide range of micronutrients. Consider supplementing with a high-quality multivitamin if you struggle to meet your needs through food alone.

Hydration is another crucial aspect of nutrition that often goes overlooked. Water is essential for regulating body temperature, transporting nutrients, and removing waste products. Aim to drink at least half your body weight in ounces of water per day, and more if you engage in intense exercise or live in a hot climate. Proper hydration can boost your metabolism, improve digestion, and enhance recovery after workouts.

To simplify meal planning and portion control, try the "Plate Method." Visualize your plate divided into three sections: half the plate should consist of non-starchy vegetables, one-quarter should be lean protein, and the remaining quarter should be complex carbohydrates. This balanced approach confirms that you are getting the right mix of nutrients at each meal without the need for tedious calorie counting.

When grocery shopping, navigating food labels can be overwhelming. Focus on reading the ingredient list rather than getting caught up in clever marketing claims. Choose products with whole, minimally processed ingredients and be mindful of serving sizes. Do not fall for the "health halo" effect, where foods are perceived as healthier simply because of their packaging or brand. Educate yourself on common misleading terms and prioritize whole, nutrient-dense foods whenever possible.

As the famous saying goes, "You can't out-exercise a bad diet." Your nutritional choices have a profound impact on your fitness results and overall well-being. By understanding the fundamentals of calories, macronutrients, micronutrients, hydration, and portion control, you will be empowered to make informed decisions and create a sustainable eating plan that supports your goals.

Key Takeaways:

- Calculate your ideal calorie intake based on your individual goals and characteristics.

- Find your optimal macronutrient balance of protein, carbs, and fat.

- Focus on nutrient-dense, whole-food sources of carbohydrates.

- Ensure adequate intake of essential micronutrients through a varied diet.

- Prioritize hydration for optimal metabolism and recovery.

- Use the "Plate Method" for easy meal planning and portion control.

- Navigate food labels with a critical eye and prioritize whole, minimally processed ingredients.

Chapter 4: Meal Planning and Prep for Success

Imagine waking up each morning, knowing exactly what delicious, nutritious meals await you throughout the day. Visualize yourself efficiently gliding through the grocery store, confidently selecting ingredients that align with your fitness goals. Envision a fridge stocked with pre-prepared, healthy dishes, ready to be enjoyed at a moment's notice.

This chapter will guide you through the process of creating a sustainable 90-day meal plan, tailored to your unique preferences and lifestyle, setting you up for success on your transformative journey. The key to staying on track with your nutrition comes from planning and preparation. By dedicating time each week to map out your meals, you will eliminate the stress and uncertainty that often leads to poor food choices.

Start by considering your favorite healthy foods and recipes and build your meal plan around them. Incorporate a variety of colorful fruits and vegetables, lean proteins, whole grains, and healthy fats to ensure you are nourishing your body with the nutrients it needs to thrive. When it is time to hit the grocery store, arm yourself with a well-organized list based on your meal plan. This will help you stay focused and avoid impulse purchases that could derail your progress.

Opt for whole, unprocessed foods whenever possible, and do not be afraid to experiment with new ingredients that align with your goals. Remember, your grocery cart should reflect the vibrant, energized life you are working towards. To streamline your meal prep process, dedicate a few hours each week to batch cooking. By preparing larger quantities of staple ingredients like grilled chicken, roasted vegetables, and quinoa, you will have the building blocks for quick, healthy meals at your fingertips. Invest in quality storage containers to keep your pre-prepped ingredients fresh and easily accessible.

To best set up your week, make a list of easy-to-prepare recipes for breakfast, lunch, dinner, and snacks. These recipes should be designed to keep you feeling satisfied and energized, while supporting your fitness goals. From protein-packed smoothie bowls to colorful stir-fries and hearty salads, you will discover that healthy eating can be both enjoyable and rewarding.

As you start on your 90-day transformation, it is crucial to develop strategies for dealing with cravings and emotional eating. When temptation strikes, pause and reflect on your goals and the reasons behind your desire to eat. Practice mindfulness techniques, such as deep breathing or meditation, to help you navigate these challenging moments. Remember, progress is not about perfection, but rather about making consistent, positive choices that align with your values.

Eating out and social situations can be particularly challenging when you are working towards a fitness goal. Yet, with a bit of planning and assertiveness, you can stay on track without sacrificing your social life. Research restaurant menus ahead of time, and do not be afraid to make special requests or modifications to ensure your meal aligns with your plan. When attending social gatherings, offer to bring a healthy dish to share, so you know there will be at least one option that supports your goals.

Finally, it is essential to approach your nutrition plan with flexibility and self-compassion. The "Flexible Five" approach allows you to incorporate small treats or indulgences into your plan without derailing your progress. By giving yourself permission to enjoy these treats in moderation, you will be less likely to feel deprived or resentful of your healthy lifestyle. As the renowned nutritionist Adelle Davis once said, "We are indeed much more than what we eat, but what we eat can nevertheless help us to be much more than what we are." By embracing the power of meal planning and preparation, you will be well on your way to becoming the best version of yourself.

Chapter 5: Supercharging Fat Loss: Advanced Strategies

Shedding those last few stubborn pounds can be frustrating, but with the right strategies, you can supercharge your fat loss and achieve the lean, toned physique you have been working towards. In this chapter, we will dive into the science of fat burning and explore advanced techniques to help you target problem areas, optimize your sleep and stress levels, and make informed decisions about fasting and supplementation. Take note of certain steps to make sure you will keep your optimal self-journey moving forward.

It is essential to understand how your body burns fat. When you create a calorie deficit by consuming fewer calories than you burn, your body uses its fat stores for energy. However, not all fat is created equal. Stubborn fat, particularly around the belly, thighs, and arms, can be more challenging to lose because of hormonal and genetic factors. To target these areas, incorporate exercises that engage multiple muscle groups and boost your metabolism. Compound movements like squats, lunges, and push-ups are excellent choices. High-intensity interval training (HIIT) is also effective for burning fat, as it keeps your metabolism elevated long after your workout ends.

Sleep plays a crucial role in fat loss, as it helps regulate hormones that control hunger and metabolism. Aim for 7-9 hours of quality sleep each night. Establish a consistent sleep schedule, create a relaxing bedtime routine, and ensure your bedroom is cool, dark, and quiet.

Stress management is another key factor in fat loss. When you are stressed, your body releases cortisol, a hormone that can lead to increased belly fat storage. Incorporate stress-reducing techniques like meditation, deep breathing, yoga, or engaging in hobbies you enjoy.

Intermittent fasting has gained popularity as a fat loss strategy, but is it right for you? Fasting involves restricting your eating to a specific window of time each day, typically 8-10 hours. While some people find success with this approach, it is not for everyone. If you have a history of disordered eating or a medical condition, discuss with your healthcare provider before trying intermittent fasting.

When it comes to supplements, be cautious. While some supplements like caffeine, green tea extract, and conjugated linoleic acid (CLA) may aid fat loss, many products make exaggerated claims and can be harmful. Focus on getting your nutrients from whole foods and ask with a registered dietitian before adding any supplements to your routine.

Finally, do not overlook the importance of gut health in weight loss. A healthy gut microbiome can improve digestion, reduce inflammation, and regulate appetite. Incorporate probiotic-rich foods like yogurt, kefir, sauerkraut, and kimchi into your diet, and consider taking a high-quality probiotic supplement.

"The key to success is to focus on goals, not obstacles." – Unknown. As you implement these advanced fat loss strategies, remember to be patient and consistent. Continue to celebrate your success and find ways to maintain momentum and motivation.

Chapter 6: Building Lean Muscle Mass in 90 Days

You have been hitting the gym consistently, pushing yourself harder each session, but you are not seeing the muscle gains you desire. Building lean muscle mass is a science, and once you understand the key principles, you can reach your body's full potential. In this chapter, we will take a close look at the biology of muscle growth, the most effective exercises for each muscle group, and the nutrition and recovery strategies that will take your physique to the next level.

The foundation of muscle growth comes from the concept of progressive overload. When you challenge your muscles with resistance training, you create microscopic tears in the muscle fibers. During the recovery process, your body repairs these tears, making the muscles stronger and larger. To keep this process going, you need to consistently increase the demand on your muscles, either by lifting heavier weights, performing more reps, or reducing rest periods between sets.

To maximize muscle activation and growth, it is crucial to focus on compound exercises that target many muscle groups simultaneously. For the chest, nothing beats the classic bench press. When performed with proper form, this exercise engages the pectoral muscles and the triceps and shoulders. Similarly, squats are the king of leg exercises, hitting the quadriceps, hamstrings, and glutes in one powerful movement. Deadlifts, rows, and overhead presses round out the essential exercises for a well-rounded muscle-building routine.

Proper form is paramount when it comes to building muscle effectively and safely. Take the time to learn the correct technique for each exercise, focusing on controlled movements and a full range of motion. Engage your core throughout each lift to maintain stability and protect your spine. When performing isolation exercises like bicep curls or leg extensions, concentrate on the mind-muscle connection, actively squeezing the targeted muscle at the peak of each contraction.

Nutrition plays a vital role in supporting muscle growth. To build lean mass, you need to consume a caloric surplus, meaning you take in more calories than you burn. However, the quality of those calories matters. Focus on lean protein sources like chicken, fish, and lean beef to provide the building blocks for muscle repair and growth. Complex carbohydrates such as brown rice, quinoa, and sweet potatoes offer sustained energy for intense workouts. Do not forget about healthy fats like avocados, nuts, and olive oil, which support hormone production and overall health.

Combine progressive overload, compound exercises, proper form, and a balanced muscle-building diet to maximize your gains. Studies have shown that consuming a protein-rich meal or shake within 30 minutes of finishing your workout can enhance muscle protein synthesis, the process by which your body builds new muscle tissue. Aim for a protein intake of 1.6 to 2.2 grams per kilogram of body weight daily, spread out over several meals. This ensures a steady supply of amino acids for your muscles throughout the day.

Real-life examples of successful muscle-building transformations abound. Take the case of John, a 35-year-old office worker who committed to a 90-day muscle-building program. By focusing on compound lifts, progressively increasing his weights, and dialing in his nutrition, John gained 12 pounds of lean muscle mass while reducing his body fat percentage from 18% to 12%. His success story highlights the power of consistency, dedication, and adherence to proven muscle-building principles.

Rest and recovery are just as important as the time you spend in the gym. During sleep, your body releases growth hormone and testosterone, two key hormones that support muscle growth and repair. Aim for 7-9 hours of quality sleep each night and consider incorporating rest days or active recovery sessions like yoga or light cardio to promote optimal recovery between workouts. Give your muscles the rest and nutrients they need to grow stronger and bigger.

Even with a well-designed program, you might come across plateaus along your muscle-building journey. When this happens, it is time to introduce advanced training techniques to shock your muscles into new growth. Techniques like drop sets, where you perform a set to failure and then immediately reduce the weight and continue for additional reps, can help push past sticking points. Supersets, which involve performing two exercises back-to-back with no rest in between, can increase workout intensity and stimulate muscle growth.

For those looking to simultaneously build muscle and lose fat, the concept of body recomposition comes into play. By carefully manipulating your calorie intake and macronutrient ratios, you can create an environment that supports muscle growth while encouraging fat loss. This approach requires a more precise tracking of your food intake and a well-structured training program that prioritizes compound lifts and high-intensity interval training (HIIT).

Key Takeaway: Advanced techniques and body recomposition strategies can help you break through plateaus and achieve your ideal physique.

- Progressive overload is the key to continuous muscle growth

- Compound exercises offer the most bang for your buck

- Proper form and mind-muscle connection enhance muscle activation

- A caloric surplus and adequate protein intake support muscle gain

- Rest and recovery are essential for muscle repair and growth

- Advanced techniques can help break through plateaus

- Body recomposition allows for simultaneous muscle gain and fat loss

Building lean muscle mass in 90 days is achievable with the right combination of training, nutrition, and recovery strategies.

Fascinating Facts:

- The average person has around 650 skeletal muscles in her body

- Muscle tissue accounts for approximately 40% of total body weight

- One pound of muscle burns around 6 calories per day at rest, compared to 2 calories for fat

- The largest muscle in the human body is the gluteus maximus (buttocks)

To put your newfound knowledge into action, follow these steps:

1. Design a workout program that focuses on compound exercises and progressive overload

2. Perfect your form for each exercise, prioritizing safety and muscle activation

3. Calculate your daily caloric and macronutrient needs for muscle gain

4. Plan and prepare meals that support your muscle-building goals

5. Prioritize rest and recovery, aiming for 7-9 hours of sleep per night

Chapter 7: Boosting Cardiovascular Health and Endurance

Imagine a life where you can efficiently climb stairs, run to catch a bus, or play with your children without getting winded. This is the power of a strong, healthy cardiovascular system. By focusing on boosting your cardiovascular health and endurance, you gain access to possibilities and improve your overall well-being.

To achieve this, it is essential to understand the different types of cardio and their unique benefits. Steady-state cardio, such as jogging or cycling, helps build a strong foundation of endurance. High-intensity interval training (HIIT) alternates between intense bursts of activity and short recovery periods, pushing your heart and lungs to their limits and burning calories efficiently. Functional movements, like squats and lunges, mimic real-world activities and improve your body's ability to handle everyday challenges.

Designing a progressive cardio plan is key to success. Start with a comfortable level of intensity and gradually increase the duration and frequency of your workouts. Aim for a mix of steady-state cardio and HIIT to reap the most cardiovascular benefits. Remember to listen to your body and allow for adequate rest and recovery between sessions.

As you advance in your cardiovascular journey, incorporate interval training to take your fitness to the next level. Alternate between high-intensity intervals and active recovery periods to challenge your heart and lungs, forcing them to adapt and grow stronger. This type of training boosts your endurance and improves your body's ability to use oxygen efficiently.

The secret to harnessing your cardiovascular potential comes from pushing your limits and embracing the power of interval training. Proper breathing techniques are essential for enhancing endurance and performance. Focus on taking deep, controlled breaths from your diaphragm, allowing your lungs to fully expand and contract. This maximizes oxygen intake and helps you maintain a steady rhythm during your workouts. Practice breathing exercises regularly to strengthen your respiratory muscles and improve your overall lung capacity.

Monitoring your heart rate is a valuable tool for tracking your progress and ensuring you are working at the right intensity. Use a heart rate watch or learn to take your pulse manually to determine your heart rate zones. Aim to exercise within your target heart rate zone, which is typically 50-85% of your maximum heart rate, depending on your fitness level and goals. By staying within these zones, you improve your cardiovascular training and avoid overexertion.

The benefits of improved cardiovascular health extend far beyond the gym. With a stronger heart and lungs, you will experience increased energy levels, better sleep, reduced stress, and improved mental clarity. Your body will be better equipped to handle the demands of daily life, allowing you to tackle challenges with confidence and resilience.

"The greatest wealth is health." - Virgil

Key Takeaways:

- Incorporate a mix of steady-state cardio, HIIT, and functional movements for optimal cardiovascular health.

- Design a progressive cardio plan that gradually increases in intensity and duration.

- Embrace interval training to push your limits and maximize cardiovascular benefits.

- Practice proper breathing techniques to enhance endurance and performance.

- Monitor your heart rate and stay within your target heart rate zones for effective training.

- Improved cardiovascular health leads to increased energy, better sleep, reduced stress, and improved overall well-being.

Chapter 8: Flexibility, Mobility, and Injury Prevention

In your pursuit of optimal fitness, you may have focused primarily on building strength and endurance, but have you given enough attention to flexibility and mobility? These often-overlooked aspects of fitness play a crucial role in enhancing your overall performance and preventing injuries. By incorporating targeted stretching routines, mind-body practices, and corrective exercises into your fitness regimen, you can perform to your body's full potential and bulletproof yourself against common setbacks.

Flexibility is about more than just being able to touch your toes or perform impressive yoga poses – it involves maintaining a healthy range of motion in your joints and muscles. When your body is flexible, you can move more efficiently, generate more power, and reduce the risk of strains and sprains. Neglecting flexibility training can lead to muscle imbalances, poor posture, and a higher likelihood of injury.

To optimize your flexibility and prepare your body for the demands of your workouts, dynamic stretching is a must. Unlike static stretching, which involves holding a stretch for an extended period, dynamic stretching involves controlled movements that mimic the exercises you will be performing. By gradually increasing your range of motion and activating your muscles, you will be primed for peak performance and less prone to injury.

While dynamic stretching is ideal for pre-workout preparation, static stretching still has its place in your fitness routine. After a challenging workout, taking the time to hold stretches for 15-30 seconds can help reduce muscle tension, promote relaxation, and improve overall flexibility. Static stretching is particularly beneficial for targeting tight muscle groups and preventing the buildup of chronic tension.

In addition to traditional stretching techniques, incorporating mind-body practices like yoga and Pilates can take your flexibility and mobility to new heights. These disciplines focus on connecting your breath with movement, enhancing body awareness, and promoting a sense of calm and balance. By regularly practicing yoga or Pilates, you will improve your flexibility and develop greater core strength, postural alignment, and mental focus.

Another valuable tool in your flexibility and recovery arsenal is foam rolling and self-massage. These techniques involve using a foam roller or massage ball to apply pressure to specific muscle groups, helping to break up adhesions, increase blood flow, and promote relaxation. By spending just a few minutes each day on self-massage, you can significantly reduce muscle soreness, improve tissue quality, and speed up your recovery between workouts.

Flexibility and mobility are essential components of a well-rounded fitness routine, contributing to improved performance, reduced injury risk, and faster recovery. While stretching and self-massage are important for maintaining flexibility, it is also crucial to address any underlying muscle imbalances or movement dysfunctions that may be holding you back. Common issues like rounded shoulders, anterior pelvic tilt, or tight hip flexors can lead to poor movement patterns and increased strain on your joints and muscles. By incorporating corrective exercises into your routine, you can target these imbalances and restore optimal function.

For example, if you spend long hours sitting at a desk, you may develop tight hip flexors and weak glutes, which can contribute to lower back pain and reduced power output in your lower body exercises. By performing targeted stretches for your hip flexors and strengthening exercises for your glutes, such as bridges or clamshells, you can correct this imbalance and improve your overall movement quality.

To take your injury prevention efforts to the next level, consider adopting a "Prehab Protocol" – a proactive approach to strengthening and conditioning your body to withstand the demands of your chosen activities. This may involve incorporating specific exercises to strengthen commonly injured areas like the shoulders, knees, or ankles, as well as focusing on proper form and technique in all your movements.

Addressing muscle imbalances and movement dysfunctions through corrective exercises and a proactive "Prehab Protocol" can help you avoid common injuries and perform at your best.

Evidence supporting the importance of flexibility and mobility in fitness is abundant. A study published in the Journal of Strength and Conditioning Research found that a 10-week stretching program significantly improved flexibility and range of motion in athletes, leading to enhanced performance and reduced injury risk. Another study in the International Journal of Sports Physical Therapy highlighted the effectiveness of foam rolling in reducing muscle soreness and improving recovery after intense exercise.

Real-life examples of athletes prioritizing flexibility and mobility are plentiful. Olympic gymnast Simone Biles, known for her incredible power and agility, credits her success partly to her dedication to stretching and mobility work. Similarly, NFL quarterback Tom Brady has emphasized the importance of pliability and flexibility in his training, allowing him to perform at an elite level well into his 40s.

As the renowned martial artist Bruce Lee once said, "Notice that the stiffest tree is most easily cracked, while the bamboo or willow survives by bending with the wind." This quote beautifully encapsulates the value of flexibility in fitness and in life. By cultivating a supple and resilient body, you will be better equipped to handle the physical and mental challenges that come your way.

Incorporating flexibility and mobility training into your fitness routine is backed by scientific evidence and the experiences of successful athletes, highlighting its importance for optimal performance and longevity. Consider these eye-opening facts and statistics:

- Over 50% of adults experience lower back pain, often due to poor flexibility and weak core muscles.

- Tight hip flexors, a common issue among sedentary people, can lead to a 30% reduction in gluteus maximus activation during exercise.

- Regular stretching can improve circulation, increasing blood flow to muscles by up to 30%.

- Foam rolling has been shown to increase range of motion by up to 10 degrees after just one session.

Key Takeaway: Neglecting flexibility and mobility can have far-reaching consequences for your health and performance, while prioritizing these aspects can yield significant benefits. To start incorporating flexibility and mobility training into your routine, follow these action steps:

1. Begin each workout with a dynamic stretching routine, focusing on the muscle groups you will be using in your exercises.

2. Perform movements like leg swings, arm circles, and walking lunges for 5-10 minutes.

3. After your workouts, spend 10-15 minutes on static stretching, holding each stretch for 15-30 seconds.

4. Target major muscle groups like your hamstrings, quadriceps, hip flexors, and chest.

5. Incorporate foam rolling or self-massage into your daily routine, spending 1-2 minutes on each major muscle group.

6. Focus on areas that feel tight or tender, breathing deeply and allowing the muscle to relax.

7. Attend a yoga or Pilates class at least once a week to improve your flexibility, core strength, and body awareness. If you cannot attend a class, follow along with online videos or practice a few basic poses at home.

8. Identify any muscle imbalances or movement dysfunctions you may have and incorporate corrective exercises into your routine.

9. Consult with a qualified fitness professional or physical therapist for guidance on specific exercises to address your individual needs.

10. Develop a "Prehab Protocol" for your specific fitness goals, incorporating exercises that target commonly injured areas and focusing on proper form and technique.

Chapter 9: Nutrition Deep Dive: Fueling Your Transformation

You have been putting in the work, hitting the gym consistently, and pushing your limits. But have you given your nutrition the same level of attention? What you eat plays a crucial role in your fitness journey, and understanding the intricacies of nutrition can take your results to the next level.

Protein is the building block of muscle, and consuming enough of it is essential for muscle growth and recovery. Aim for a minimum of 0.8 grams per pound of body weight, spread out over several meals throughout the day. High-quality sources like lean meats, fish, eggs, and plant-based options like tofu and legumes should be staples in your diet.

Carbohydrates are your body's primary energy source, and timing them correctly can make a significant difference in your performance. Focus on consuming complex carbs like whole grains, fruits, and vegetables throughout the day. Consider adding a quick-digesting carb source like a banana or rice cakes before and after your workouts for an extra energy boost.

Healthy fats are often overlooked, but they play a vital role in hormone production and overall health. Incorporate sources like avocados, nuts, seeds, and fatty fish into your meals to confirm you are getting enough of these essential nutrients. Do not be afraid of fat – it will not make you fat when consumed in moderation.

Your pre- and post-workout nutrition can make or break your results. Aim to have a balanced meal containing protein and carbs 1-2 hours before your workout and follow up with a protein and carb-rich meal within an hour of finishing your session. This will help fuel your performance and kickstart the recovery process.

Detoxes and cleanses have gained popularity in recent years, but the reality is that most of them are ineffective and unsustainable. Your body is equipped with its own detoxification system. The best way to support it is by eating a balanced diet rich in whole foods, staying hydrated, and limiting your intake of processed junk.

If you have dietary restrictions, such as following a vegan or gluten-free diet, it is important to plan your meals carefully to confirm you're getting all the necessary nutrients. Focus on a variety of whole foods and consider working with a registered dietitian to create a personalized plan that meets your needs. Make sure to stick to the plan and stay the course.

Supplements can be a useful addition to your nutrition plan, but they should never replace a balanced diet. Stick to the basics like a high-quality protein powder, creatine, and a multivitamin, and be wary of flashy marketing claims. Always talk to a healthcare professional before starting any new supplement regimen.

Nutrition is a powerful tool in your fitness arsenal. By focusing on high-quality protein, strategic carb timing, healthy fats, and proper pre- and post-workout nutrition, you can optimize your results and fuel your transformation. The evidence supporting the importance of nutrition in fitness is overwhelming. Countless studies have shown that a balanced diet rich in protein, complex carbs, and healthy fats can lead to improved performance, better recovery, and enhanced overall health. For example, a 2018 study published in the Journal of the International Society of Sports Nutrition found that consuming a protein-rich meal before and after resistance training led to increased muscle protein synthesis and improved recovery compared to a placebo.

Real-life examples of the power of nutrition are everywhere. Take the case of Sally, a busy professional who struggled to make progress in the gym despite consistent training. After working with a nutritionist to optimize her diet, she noticed a significant improvement in her energy levels, recovery time, and overall physique. By focusing on whole foods, proper macronutrient balance, and strategic meal timing, Sally was able to take her fitness to the next level.

As the famous saying goes, "You can't out-train a bad diet." No matter how hard you work in the gym, if your nutrition is not on point, you will be fighting an uphill battle. By making nutrition a priority and fueling your body with the right nutrients, you can succeed to your full potential and achieve the transformation you have been working towards.

Key Takeaway: A well-designed nutrition plan is just as important as your training program. By focusing on the key principles of protein intake, carb timing, healthy fats, and pre- and post-workout nutrition, you can optimize your results and reach your goals faster. Here are some interesting bullet points to keep in mind as you navigate your nutrition journey:

- Hydration is crucial for performance and recovery. Aim for at least 0.5-1 ounce of water per pound of body weight daily.

- Meal prepping can save you time and confirm you always have healthy options on hand.

- Do not be afraid to experiment with new foods and recipes to keep your diet interesting and enjoyable.

- Listen to your body and pay attention to how different foods make you feel. Everyone's optimal diet is unique.

Nutrition does not have to be complicated. By focusing on whole foods, staying hydrated, and being mindful of your choices, you can create a sustainable plan that supports your fitness goals and overall health. Here are some eye-opening facts and statistics that highlight the importance of nutrition in fitness:

- A study published in the Journal of the American Medical Association found that people who consumed a high-protein diet (25% of daily calories) lost 10% more belly fat than those on a low-protein diet (15% of daily calories).

- Research has shown that consuming a meal containing 20-40 grams of protein before bed can enhance muscle protein synthesis and improve recovery overnight.

- A 2019 survey by the Council for Responsible Nutrition found that 77% of U.S. Adults use dietary supplements, with the most popular being multivitamins, vitamin D, and omega-3 fatty acids.

The science behind nutrition and fitness is constantly evolving, but the core principles remain the same. By staying informed and making evidence-based choices, you can optimize your diet for most results. Now that you understand the importance of nutrition in your fitness journey, it is time to take action. Here are some specific, detailed

steps you can take to start fueling your
transformation:

1. Calculate your daily protein needs based on
    your body weight and fitness goals and plan
    your meals accordingly.

2. Incorporate a variety of complex carbs and
    healthy fats into your diet, focusing on whole
    food sources.

3. Experiment with different pre- and post-
    workout meal combinations to find what
    works best for your energy levels and
    recovery.

Chapter 10: Mind-Body Connection: Mental Strategies for Success

Your mind is your most powerful ally on the pathway to getting your fitness goals. The connection between your mental state and physical performance is undeniable, and harnessing this power can propel you to new heights. Visualization, a technique used by elite athletes and high-performers, is a key tool in your mental arsenal. By vividly imagining yourself getting your desired physique and performing at your best, you create a mental blueprint that guides your actions and decisions.

As you progress through your transformation, it is crucial to develop a positive body image. Embrace the changes you see in the mirror and celebrate the strength and capabilities of your body. Shift your focus from perceived flaws to the incredible feats your body can accomplish. Surround yourself with affirmations and reminders of your worth, and practice self-compassion when faced with setbacks or challenges.

Mindfulness and meditation are powerful practices for reducing stress and enhancing focus.

By taking a few minutes each day to quiet your mind and focus on your breath, you create a sense of calm and clarity that carries over into your workouts and daily life. Incorporate mindfulness into your fitness routine by staying present and fully engaged in each movement, as opposed to letting your mind wander or dwell on distractions.

"The mind is everything. What you think, you become." – Buddha. Mental barriers and self-sabotaging behaviors can derail even the most dedicated fitness enthusiasts. Recognize the negative thought patterns and limiting beliefs that hold you back, such as "I'm not strong enough" or "I don't have time." Challenge these thoughts with evidence of your progress and capabilities and replace them with empowering affirmations like "I am capable of achieving my goals" and "I prioritize my health and well-being."

Sleep is a critical component of both mental health and physical performance. Aim for 7-9 hours of quality sleep each night to allow your body and mind to recover, repair, and recharge. Establish a consistent sleep routine, create a relaxing bedtime environment, and avoid stimulating activities like screen time before bed. Well-rested, you will have the energy and focus to tackle your workouts and make healthier choices throughout the day.

Building resilience and grit is essential for long-term success in fitness and life. Embrace challenges as opportunities for growth, and view setbacks as temporary obstacles to overcome. Cultivate a growth mindset, believing that your abilities can be developed through dedication and hard work. Surround yourself with a supportive network of friends, family, and fitness professionals who encourage and inspire you to keep pushing forward.

The "Mental Momentum Method" is a powerful technique for pushing through tough days when motivation is low. Start by setting a small, achievable goal for your workout, such as completing the first 10 minutes or one set of each exercise. Once you achieve that goal, build on that momentum by setting another small goal, and continue this process throughout your workout. By focusing on small, incremental progress, you will build the mental toughness and discipline to overcome any obstacle.

Chapter 11: Lifestyle Integration: Making Your 90-Day Plan Sustainable

You have made incredible progress over the past few months, dedicating yourself to a healthier lifestyle and pushing your limits in the gym. As you approach the end of your 90-day journey, it is crucial to consider how you will maintain your hard-earned results and continue making fitness a priority in your life. Integrating your fitness plan into your daily routine is key to long-term success, allowing you to balance your goals with work, family, and personal commitments.

Creating a supportive environment is essential for staying on track. Surround yourself with people who understand and encourage your healthy lifestyle. Share your goals with loved ones and explain how they can help you stay accountable. If you encounter unsupportive friends or family members, remember that this is your path, and you have the right to prioritize your well-being. Gently remind them of your reasons for pursuing a healthier life and ask for their understanding and cooperation.

Balancing fitness with a busy schedule can be challenging, but it is not impossible. Start by identifying pockets of time you can dedicate to exercise, even if it's just 20-30 minutes a day. Consider waking up earlier, using your lunch break, or fitting in a quick workout before dinner. Maximize your efficiency by preparing meals in advance, packing gym bags the night before, and combining errands with exercise, such as walking or biking to the store.

When work or family obligations need travel, it is important to have strategies in place to maintain your fitness routine. Research hotels with well-equipped gyms or pack resistance bands for a quick in-room workout. Scout out local parks or trails for outdoor exercise opportunities. If dining out is inevitable, make informed choices by reviewing menus in advance and opting for grilled, baked, or roasted dishes with plenty of vegetables.

Incorporating active hobbies into your lifestyle can make fitness feel less like a chore and more like an enjoyable part of your day. Explore activities that excite you, such as hiking, dancing, rock climbing, or martial arts. Joining a recreational sports league or fitness class can provide a sense of community and accountability while keeping exercise engaging and fun.

As you continue your fitness journey, remember that rest and recovery are just as important as the time you spend in the gym. Adequate sleep, proper nutrition, and regular rest days allow your body to repair, rebuild, and come back stronger. Aim for 7-9 hours of quality sleep each night, fuel your body with whole, nutrient-dense foods, and listen to your body's signals for when it needs a break.

Sustainable fitness requires a balanced approach that prioritizes your goals while allowing flexibility for life's demands. Evidence suggests that individuals who successfully maintain long-term fat loss and fitness engage in consistent exercise routines, regularly watch their progress, and have strong social support systems. A study published in the Journal of Obesity found that participants who maintained their fat loss for over a year reported higher levels of physical activity, self-monitoring, and positive social support compared to those who regained weight.

For example, Lisa, a busy mother of two, successfully integrated her 90-day fitness plan into her lifestyle by involving her family in meal planning and preparation, scheduling her workouts during her children's sports practices, and finding an accountability partner to join her for weekly hikes. By making fitness a priority and creating a supportive environment, Lisa was able to maintain her results and continue progressing toward her long-term health goals.

"The only limit to your impact is your imagination and commitment." - Tony Robbins.

Analyzing your 90-day fitness journey can provide valuable insights for long-term success. Reflect on the strategies that worked well for you, such as meal prepping, scheduling workouts, or finding a workout buddy. Identify areas where you struggled, like late-night snacking or skipping workouts because of fatigue, and brainstorm solutions to overcome these challenges in the future. By understanding your strengths and weaknesses, you can develop a personalized plan for sustainable fitness.

A study conducted by the National Weight Control Registry found that individuals who successfully maintained significant fat loss for over a year shared common habits, such as:

- Eating breakfast regularly

- Engaging in high levels of physical activity (about 1 hour per day)

- Weighing themselves weekly

- Watching less than 10 hours of TV per week

- Maintaining a consistent eating pattern across weekdays and weekends

Key Takeaway: Adopting healthy habits and creating a supportive environment are crucial for long-term fitness success.

- Surround yourself with people who support and encourage your healthy lifestyle

- Incorporate physical activity into your daily routine, even in small increments

- Plan ahead for meals, workouts, and travel to stay on track

- Find active hobbies that make fitness enjoyable and engaging

- Prioritize rest and recovery to prevent burnout and maintain progress

- Small, consistent actions lead to significant results over time.

- 75% of successful weight maintainers eat breakfast every day

- People who track their food intake are more likely to maintain fat loss

- Individuals who exercise for an hour or more daily are more successful at keeping weight off

Your 90-day plan is just the beginning of a lifelong journey toward better health and well-being.

Specific Action Steps:

1. Schedule a weekly planning session to review your upcoming commitments and prioritize your workouts and meal preparation.

2. Identify three active hobbies or activities you enjoy and commit to engaging in them at least once a week.

3. Have an open conversation with your loved ones about your fitness goals and how they can support you in maintaining a healthy lifestyle.

Chapter 12: Tracking Progress and Adjusting Your Plan

"The only way to keep your health is to eat what you don't want, drink what you don't like, and do what you'd rather not." - Mark Twain

As you begin on your fitness and nutrition journey, it is crucial to understand that progress goes beyond the numbers on the scale. Comprehensive progress tracking is your under-the-radar advantage to stay motivated, make informed decisions, and achieve long-lasting results. Embrace the power of progress photos, measurements, and fitness tests. These tools provide a more complete picture of your transformation than weight alone. Progress photos visually showcase your changing body composition, while measurements reveal inch loss in specific areas. Fitness tests, such as strength assessments or cardiovascular endurance challenges, demonstrate your improving physical capabilities. When it comes to body fat measurement, navigate the options wisely. Skinfold calipers, bioelectrical impedance scales, and hydrostatic weighing each have their pros and cons.

Consistency in the method you choose is key for accurate comparisons over time. Remember, body fat percentage is just one piece of the puzzle. As you gather data, be prepared to adjust your plan based on results. If progress stalls, it's time to reassess your strategies. Plateaus are a normal part of the process, but they don't have to derail your success. Experiment with variables such as calorie intake, macronutrient ratios, exercise intensity, or training frequency to reignite progress. Small tweaks can lead to significant breakthroughs.

Amidst the focus on quantitative measures, do not overlook the importance of non-scale victories. Celebrate the increased energy, improved sleep, clearer skin, and enhanced confidence that come with your healthier lifestyle. These qualitative markers of progress are powerful motivators that keep you committed to your goals. To streamline your progress tracking, create a personal dashboard that combines many metrics. Include body measurements, fitness test results, daily nutrition logs, and subjective assessments of well-being. This holistic approach paints a comprehensive picture of your progress and helps you identify patterns and correlations.

Progress tracking is a multifaceted endeavor that goes beyond the scale. Embrace a comprehensive approach to assess your transformation and make informed adjustments to your plan. Remember, progress is rarely linear. Expect fluctuations and plateaus as part of the process. Trust in the added effect of your consistent efforts. By regularly monitoring your progress through many lenses, you arm yourself with the insights needed to make strategic adjustments and maintain forward momentum. By mastering the art of progress tracking, you equip yourself with the tools to navigate the ups and downs of your fitness and nutrition journey.

Key Takeaways:

- Utilize progress photos, measurements, and fitness tests for a comprehensive assessment

- Choose a consistent body fat measurement method and interpret results in context

- Adjust your plan based on results, experimenting with variables to overcome plateaus

- Celebrate non-scale victories as powerful motivators

- Create a personal progress dashboard integrating many metrics

- Embrace the non-linear nature of progress and trust the process

Chapter 13: Special Considerations for Different Populations

"The greatest wealth is health." - Virgil

As you set off on your fitness and nutrition journey, it is crucial to understand that one size does not fit all. Your age, lifestyle, health conditions, and unique circumstances play a significant role in shaping your approach to wellness. In this chapter, we will explore how to adapt the 90-day plan to meet the specific needs of various populations, ensuring that everyone can achieve their goals safely and effectively.

For seniors, the focus should be on functional fitness and maintaining bone health. Incorporate exercises that mimic everyday movements, such as squats, lunges, and balance drills, to improve overall mobility and reduce the risk of falls. Resistance training is essential for preventing age-related muscle loss and osteoporosis. Aim for two to three strength sessions per week, using lighter weights and higher repetitions to minimize joint stress.

New mothers face unique challenges when it comes to postpartum fitness. Before diving into any exercise routine, ask your healthcare provider to confirm that you're cleared for physical activity. Start with gentle exercises like walking, pelvic floor exercises, and core strengthening moves. Gradually increase the intensity and duration of your workouts as your body recovers. Remember to listen to your body and prioritize rest and recovery.

If you are managing a chronic condition, such as diabetes or heart disease, diet and exercise can be powerful tools for improving your health. Work closely with your healthcare team to develop a personalized plan that takes your specific needs into account. Focus on nutrient-dense, whole foods and engage in regular, moderate-intensity exercise to help control symptoms and reduce the risk of complications.

Shift workers and those with irregular schedules may find it challenging to maintain a consistent fitness routine. The key is to prioritize exercise whenever possible, even if it means breaking up your workouts into shorter sessions throughout the day. Meal prepping and keeping healthy snacks on hand can help you stay on track with your nutrition goals, despite unconventional work hours.

Your body type and genetic factors can influence how you respond to different diet and exercise strategies. Ectomorphs, who tend to be naturally lean, may need to focus on calorie-dense foods and strength training to build muscle mass. Endomorphs, who have a higher body fat percentage, may benefit from a lower-carb diet and high-intensity interval training (HIIT) to boost metabolism. Mesomorphs, with their naturally athletic build, can thrive on a balanced diet and a variety of exercises.

Hormonal changes, such as those experienced during menopause and andropause, can impact your fitness progress. For women going through menopause, prioritize weight-bearing exercises to maintain bone density and consider incorporating yoga or Pilates to manage stress and improve flexibility. Men experiencing andropause may benefit from exercises that boost testosterone, such as compound lifts and HIIT.

If you have limited mobility or chronic pain, modifications to the 90-day plan may be necessary. Work with a qualified fitness professional or physical therapist to develop a program that accommodates your limitations. Low-impact exercises like swimming, cycling, and yoga can provide a great workout without exacerbating pain or discomfort. Focus on proper form and technique to minimize the risk of injury.

Chapter 14: The Role of Technology in Your 90-Day Journey

In today's digital age, technology has become an integral part of our lives, and your 90-day fitness journey is no exception. From wearable devices to mobile apps and virtual coaching, the right tech tools can help you stay motivated, track your progress, and achieve your goals more efficiently. In this chapter, we will explore how you can leverage technology to supercharge your transformation and make the most of your 90-day journey.

When it comes to choosing a fitness tracker or smartwatch, it is essential to consider your specific goals and needs. If you are primarily focused on cardio and step counting, a basic fitness tracker with heart rate monitoring might suffice. However, if you are engaging in a variety of workouts and want more advanced features like GPS tracking, sleep monitoring, and smartphone notifications, a smartwatch could be a better investment. Take the time to research and compare different devices to find one that aligns with your preferences and budget.

In addition to wearables, there is a plethora of apps and software designed to simplify meal planning and tracking. These tools allow you to log your food intake, monitor your macronutrient ratios, and even generate personalized meal plans based on your goals and dietary preferences. Some popular options include MyFitnessPal, LoseIt!, and Noom. By consistently tracking your nutrition, you will gain a better understanding of your eating habits and be able to make informed decisions to support your progress.

As you start on your 90-day journey, you might also consider exploring virtual personal training or online coaching. These services connect you with experienced fitness professionals who can provide customized workout plans, form corrections, and accountability check-ins, all from the comfort of your own home. Platforms like Trainerize, Future, and OpenFit offer a range of coaching options to suit different budgets and preferences. With the guidance of a virtual coach, you can confirm that you're following a safe and effective program tailored to your unique needs.

Social media can also be a powerful tool for accountability and support throughout your 90-day transformation. By connecting with like-minded people or joining online fitness communities, you can share your progress, exchange tips and encouragement, and stay motivated when the going gets tough. Platforms like Instagram, Facebook, and Reddit host a variety of fitness-focused groups and challenges that can help you stay engaged and inspired. Just be mindful of the potential pitfalls of social media, such as comparison traps and information overload, and focus on using these platforms in a way that uplifts and empowers you.

In recent years, AI-powered fitness plans have gained popularity, promising personalized workout recommendations based on your fitness level, goals, and preferences. While these algorithms can be helpful in providing structure and variety to your workouts, it is important to approach them with a critical eye. AI-generated plans may not always take into account your person limitations, injuries, or equipment access, so it's crucial to listen to your body and make modifications as needed. If you do choose to use an AI-powered plan, consider it a starting point as opposed to a rigid prescription, and do not hesitate to talk to a human expert if you have concerns or questions.

Technology can also be a valuable ally in ensuring proper form and technique during your workouts. Apps like Onyx and Kaia use your smartphone camera to analyze your movements and provide real-time feedback on your form. This can be especially helpful if you are new to certain exercises or do not have access to in-person coaching. However, keep in mind that these apps are not foolproof and should be used in conjunction with other resources like instructional videos and professional guidance to minimize the risk of injury.

As you combine technology into your 90-day journey, it is crucial to consider the privacy implications of the tools you use. Many fitness apps and devices collect personal data such as your location, heart rate, and sleep patterns, which can be valuable to advertisers and other third parties. Before committing to a particular platform, take the time to review its privacy policy and understand how your data will be used and shared. Opt for apps and devices that prioritize user privacy and offer robust security features like two-factor authentication and data encryption.

Technology can be a powerful ally in your 90-day transformation, but it is essential to use it mindfully and in alignment with your personal goals and values. One study published in the Journal of Medical Internet Research found that participants who used a fitness app with gamification features like points and rewards were more likely to maintain their physical activity levels over time compared to those who used a non-gamified app. This suggests that incorporating elements of fun and competition into your fitness tech stack can help keep you engaged and motivated throughout your progress. An example of the power of technology in fitness is the success story of Jerry, a 45-year-old father of two who used a combination of a smartwatch, a nutrition tracking app, and virtual coaching to lose 50 pounds and reverse his type 2 diabetes. By leveraging these tools to stay accountable and make informed lifestyle choices, Jerry was able to transform his health and quality of life in just 90 days.

As the renowned fitness expert Jillian Michaels once said, "Technology is a tool that can help you achieve your goals, but it's not a magic bullet. You still have to put in the work and make the right choices every day." When analyzing the role of technology in your 90-day journey, it is clear that it can be a valuable asset, but it's not a one-size-fits-all solution. The key is to find the tools that resonate with your personality, lifestyle, and goals, and to use them in a way that supports as opposed to replaces your own intuition and effort. By striking the right balance between technology and personal accountability, you can create a powerful synergy that propels you towards your desired transformation.

The most effective approach to fitness technology is one that combines the best of both worlds: the efficiency and insights of digital tools with the wisdom and adaptability of human intuition. A study by the University of South Australia found that fitness apps that incorporate social features like leaderboards and challenges can increase physical activity levels by up to 35%. The global market for fitness apps is expected to reach $14.7 billion by 2026, with a compound annual growth rate of 23.5% from 2020 to 2026 . The fitness technology landscape is constantly evolving, and by staying informed and adaptable, you can harness its power to support your 90-day transformation and beyond.

As you start on your technology-enhanced fitness journey, here are some specific action steps to consider:

1. Research and invest in a fitness tracker or smartwatch that aligns with your goals and preferences, taking into account factors like battery life, water resistance, and app compatibility.

2. Experiment with different nutrition tracking apps to find one that is user-friendly and comprehensive and make a habit of logging your meals and snacks consistently.

3. Explore virtual coaching options and take advantage of free trials or introductory offers to find a platform and coach that resonates with your personality and goals.

4. Join online fitness communities or challenges that align with your interests and values, and

engage regularly by sharing your progress, asking questions, and supporting others.

5. When using AI-powered fitness plans, approach them with a critical eye and be prepared to make modifications based on your body's feedback and personal limitations.

6. Incorporate form-checking apps or videos into your workout routine and seek out human guidance from a qualified fitness professional to confirm you're using proper technique.

Chapter 15: Beyond 90 Days: Maintaining Your Transformation

"Success is the sum of small efforts, repeated day in and day out." - Robert Collier

Congratulations! You have made it through your 90-day transformation, and the results are undeniable. Your body is stronger, leaner, and healthier than ever before. But now that you have reached this milestone, you might be wondering, "What's next?" maintaining your hard-earned progress needs a shift in mindset and a commitment to sustainable lifestyle habits. As you transition from a structured plan to a more flexible approach, it is essential to develop strategies that will keep you motivated without the urgency of a specific end date. One effective method is to set new goals and challenges that excite you. Whether it is training for a 5K race, mastering a new yoga pose, or trying a new healthy recipe each week, having fresh goals will keep your fitness journey engaging and rewarding.

The "Lifestyle Integration Method" is a powerful tool for creating permanent change. This approach involves gradually incorporating healthy habits into your daily routine until they become second nature. For example, instead of viewing exercise as a chore, make it a non-negotiable part of your day, just like brushing your teeth. By seamlessly integrating these practices into your life, you will find it easier to maintain your transformation for the long haul.

When it comes to nutrition, it is crucial to adjust your plan to support your new goals. If you're aiming to maintain your current physique, you may need to slightly increase your calorie intake to find your maintenance level. On the other hand, if you are looking to continue making progress, you will need to fine-tune your macronutrient ratios and ensure that you are fueling your body with the right nutrients to support your training.

The importance of periodization in long-term fitness plans cannot be overstated. Periodization involves strategically varying your workouts over time to prevent plateaus and improve results. By cycling through phases of intensity, volume, and recovery, you will keep your body challenged and avoid burnout. This approach also allows you to target specific areas of improvement, such as strength, endurance, or flexibility, depending on your goals.

Despite your best efforts, setbacks are an inevitable part of any fitness journey. The key is to develop resilience and learn to get back on track quickly. If you miss a workout or indulge in an unhealthy meal, do not beat yourself up. Instead, thank the slip-up, and recommit to your goals with renewed determination. Remember, progress isn't always linear, and small missteps do not define your overall success. As you begin this new phase of your fitness journey, embrace the power of consistency and patience. Sustainable change takes time, but by focusing on progress over perfection, you will continue to see results and feel the benefits of a healthy lifestyle.

Key Takeaways:

- Set new goals and challenges to maintain motivation

- Use the "Lifestyle Integration Method" for permanent change

- Adjust your nutrition plan to support your new goals

- Incorporate periodization to prevent plateaus and improve results

- Develop resilience to deal with setbacks and stay on track

- Embrace consistency and patience for sustainable, long-term success

By implementing these strategies and maintaining a positive mindset, you will preserve your 90-day transformation and continue to grow and thrive in your fitness journey.

Appendix A: Quick Reference 90-Day Workout Plans for Different Goals

Embarking on a 90-day workout plan is an exciting experience that can reshape your body and elevate your fitness to new heights. Whether you are aiming to build muscle, lose fat, or improve overall conditioning, a well-structured plan is essential for success. In this chapter, we will briefly explore a variety of 90-day workout plans tailored to different goals, empowering you to choose the path that aligns with your aspirations.

As the renowned bodybuilder and actor Arnold Schwarzenegger once said, "The last three or four reps is what makes the muscle grow. This area of pain divides a champion from someone who is not a champion." Embrace the challenge and push yourself beyond your perceived limits, for that is where true progress lies. When selecting a 90-day workout plan, consider your current fitness level and the specific goals you wish to achieve.

LEAN MUSCLE:

For those seeking to build lean muscle mass, a plan that emphasizes progressive resistance training, targeting each major muscle group with compound exercises, is ideal. Incorporate exercises like squats, deadlifts, bench presses, and rows, gradually increasing the weight and volume over time to stimulate muscle growth.

FAT LOSS:

If fat loss is your primary goal, a plan that combines high-intensity interval training (HIIT) with strength training exercises will be your ally. HIIT workouts, such as sprints, burpees, and mountain climbers, elevate your heart rate and boost metabolism, helping you burn fat efficiently. Complement these intense sessions with resistance training to maintain and build lean muscle, which further enhances your body's fat-burning potential.

ENDURANCE:

For those aiming to improve overall conditioning and endurance, a plan that incorporates a mix of cardiovascular exercises and functional training is the way to go. Engage in activities like running, cycling, swimming, or rowing to strengthen your heart and lungs. Incorporate body weight exercises, such as push-ups, pull-ups, and lunges, to develop functional strength and improve your body's ability to handle everyday tasks with ease.

Regardless of the plan you choose, consistency and progression are key. Start with a solid foundation and gradually increase the intensity and complexity of your workouts. Keep track of your progress, celebrate your achievements, and make adjustments as needed to ensure you're consistently moving towards your goals.

Choosing the right 90-day workout plan is crucial for accessing your fitness goals. Whether you're aiming to build muscle, lose fat, or improve overall conditioning, a tailored plan that aligns with your aspirations and current fitness level will maximize your results. As you start on your 90-day workout journey, remember to listen to your body and provide it with the necessary rest and nutrition to support your progress. Adequate sleep, a balanced diet rich in whole foods, and proper hydration are essential components of any successful fitness plan.

In bullet points, here are the key takeaways from this chapter:

- Choose a 90-day workout plan that aligns with your specific goals and current fitness level.

- Progressive resistance training is ideal for building lean muscle mass.

- High-intensity interval training (HIIT) combined with strength training promotes effective fat loss.

- A mix of cardiovascular exercises and functional training improves overall conditioning and endurance.

- Consistency, progression, and tracking your progress are crucial for success.

- Prioritize rest, nutrition, and hydration to support your fitness journey.

Appendix B: Progress Tracking Sheets and Journals

Remember, as the saying goes, "You can't manage what you don't measure."

Tracking your progress is a crucial component of attaining your fitness goals. By consistently monitoring your workouts, nutrition, and overall well-being, you gain valuable insights into what is working and what needs improvement. Tracking your progress through written journals or apps help you stay organized, motivated, and accountable throughout your fitness journey. This will allow you to visually see your progress over time, celebrating your gains and identifying areas where you may need to push yourself further. In addition to tracking your fitness, also keep a food journal to gain a better understanding of your eating habits and can make informed decisions to support your fitness goals.

By taking a holistic approach to your fitness journey, you recognize the importance of rest, recovery, and mental well-being in achieving optimal results. Record and track fitness and nutrition to establish a consistent routine of filling them out daily or after each workout. Set aside a few minutes at the end of each day to reflect on your progress and note any challenges or successes you experienced.

Over time, you will accumulate a wealth of data that can help you identify patterns, make informed adjustments, and celebrate your achievements. Remember, progress is not always linear. There may be days when you feel like you are not making the desired progress or encountering setbacks. However, by consistently tracking your progress, you will be able to see the bigger picture and recognize the overall positive trajectory of your efforts.

In addition to written tracking and/or journals of your progress, consider exploring digital tools and apps that can complement your progress monitoring. Many fitness apps offer features such as workout logging, nutrition tracking, and goal setting, making it even more convenient to stay on top of your progress.

Key Takeaways:

- Tracking your progress is essential for attaining your fitness goals.

- Use the provided workout and nutrition tracking sheets to monitor your progress consistently.

- Take a holistic approach by also tracking sleep, hydration, and stress management.

- Establish a routine of filling out the sheets daily or after each workout.

- Celebrate your achievements and use the data to make informed adjustments.

- Consider complementing your written tracking and/or journals with digital tools and apps for added convenience.

www.ingramcontent.com/pod-product-compliance
Lightning Source LLC
Chambersburg PA
CBHW061507250726
48657CB00005B/1752